Baby Shower

_____

_____

_____

_____

_____

Name	Gift

Name	Gift

Name	Gift

Name	Gift

Name	Gift

Name

Gift

Name	Gift

Name | Gift

Name	Gift

Name | Gift

www.ingramcontent.com/pod-product-compliance
Lightning Source LLC
Chambersburg PA
CBHW041653260326

41914CB00018B/1627